EMILIA DANIELS

Radiant Skin

A Comprehensive Guide Skin Care For Every Type And Condition

GOD and loved ones

Contents

Acknowledgement

Colleagues who contributed to this book. Special thanks to Mrs Chioma whose contribution was priceless

INTRODUCTION

The skin is the biggest organ of the body and plays a crucial role in protecting our internal organs from external factors such as pollutants, UV radiation, and harmful bacteria. Given its importance, it is important that we take proper care of our skin to ensure its health and longevity.

However, despite its importance, many people tend to overlook proper skincare practices. This can lead to a variety of skin issues that can range from minor irritations to severe conditions that can impact our general health and well-being.

This is where your book comes in. In this complete guide to skincare, you will learn everything you need to know to care for your skin properly. You will gain a deep understanding of the different skin types and the things that affect them. You will also learn about the common skin issues that people face and how to address them successfully.

The first chapter of the book will focus on knowing your skin type. You will learn about the five basic skin types: oily, dry, combination, sensitive, and normal, and how to decide which category your skin falls under. By understanding your skin type, you will be able to choose the right skincare products and build a daily skincare routine that caters to your specific needs.

The future chapters will delve deeper into individual skin issues and their causes. You will learn about common skin issues such as acne, rosacea, eczema, psoriasis, and aging skin, and the factors that lead to these conditions. You will also explore the different treatment choices available, including over-the-counter skincare products, prescription medications, and natural remedies.

The book will also touch on the value of healthy eating for healthy skin. You will learn about foods that promote healthy skin and the link between diet and skin problems. Additionally, you will study other factors that affect your skin, such as sun exposure, smoking, and stress.

Finally, the book will cover skincare for different stages of life, including babies, children, teenagers, pregnant women, and menopausal women. You will learn how to build a skincare routine that caters to your specific needs based on your age and gender.

In conclusion, proper skincare is important for maintaining healthy, radiant skin. With the help of this book, you will gain a deep understanding of how to care for your skin, address common skin problems, and promote overall skin health.

Understanding Your Skin Type

- The five basic skin types: oily, dry, combination, sensitive, and normal
- How to determine your skin type
- Factors that affect skin type

Knowing your skin type is the first step in creating a proper skincare routine. There are five basic types of skin: normal, combination, sensitive, oily, and dry. Every skin type has distinctive qualities and needs a different approach to skincare.

Sebum, the skin's natural oil, is produced in excess in people with oily skin. A shiny appearance and a propensity to break out can result from this. On the other hand, dry skin is characterized by a reduction in oil production, which leaves it flaky, rough, and itchy. Dry cheeks and an oily T-zone (forehead, nose, and chin) are characteristics of combination skin. External factors like fragrance, harsh ingredients, and extreme temperatures can easily irritate sensitive skin. Normal skin is well-balanced, produces sebum in a healthy amount, and has few skin problems.

Start by washing your face with a mild cleanser and patting it dry before determining your skin type. Look at your skin in the mirror and look for the following characteristics after an hour:

- **Oily skin:** Pores that are visible, a shiny appearance, and a propensity to break out.
  - **Dry skin:** Skin that is flaky, rough, itchy, and tight.
  - **Combination skin:** Dry cheeks and an oily T-zone (forehead, nose, and chin).
  - **Sensitive skin:** Itchy and red, easily irritated by environmental factors.
  - **Normal skin:** Balanced, producing a healthy amount of sebum, with few skin problems.

Once your skin type has been identified, it is critical to pick the best skincare products and create a daily skincare routine that meets your unique requirements. Pick products that are oil-free and non-comedogenic for oily skin. Look for moisturizing components like hyaluronic acid and glycerin if you have dry skin. Use skincare products for both oily and dry skin types if you have combination skin. Choose gentle products without fragrances if you have sensitive skin. Choose skincare products for normal skin that preserve the skin's natural balance.

Genetics, hormones, age, and environmental factors all influence skin type. For instance, hormonal changes during adolescence can cause oily skin, whereas aging can cause dry skin because oil production declines. Skin health can also be impacted by environmental factors such as pollution, climate, and sun exposure.

In conclusion, knowing your skin type is crucial for creating a skincare routine that is suitable for your individual requirements. You can choose the best skincare products and procedures to promote healthy, radiant skin by understanding your skin type and the factors that influence it.

Daily Skin Care Routine

- The basic steps of a daily skincare routine
- How to choose the right skincare products for your skin type
- Tips for keeping your skin healthy and glowing

Creating a daily skincare regimen is essential for preserving healthy, radiant skin. Three steps make up a standard skincare regimen: cleansing, toning, and moisturizing. The morning and evening times of the day should be used to carry out these actions.

First, clean up

In any skincare routine, cleansing comes first. It cleans the skin of dirt, oil, and impurities so that it can breathe and better absorb skincare products. Pick an appropriate gentle cleanser for your skin type. Choose a gel or foam cleanser for oily skin to help regulate oil production. Use a cream or lotion cleanser that hydrates and nourishes the skin if you have dry skin.

Phase 2: Toning

In a skincare routine, toning is an optional step. It helps to clean up any leftover dirt or impurities, balance the pH level of the skin, and get the skin ready for moisturizing. Pick a toner that's appropriate for your skin type. Use a salicylic acid or witch hazel-containing toner on oily skin to reduce sebum production. Choose a toner for dry skin that has hydrating components like aloe vera or hyaluronic acid.

Third step: moisturizing

The last step in a skincare routine is moisturizing. It keeps the skin moisturized and protected, keeping it radiant and soft. Identify the best moisturizer for your skin type. Use a thin, oil-free moisturizer that won't clog pores on oily skin. Select a rich, creamy moisturizer that offers intense hydration for dry skin.

You can incorporate additional skincare procedures into your daily routine in addition to the fundamental ones to maintain healthy, glowing skin. Here are a few advices:

1. Wear sunscreen: Use a broad-spectrum sunscreen with an SPF of at least 30 to shield your skin from the sun's damaging rays.

2. Exfoliate: By removing dead skin cells, exfoliating helps to reveal smoother, more radiant skin. Use an exfoliant once or twice a week that is appropriate for your skin type.

3. Use serums to target specific skin issues like aging, hyperpigmentation, and acne. Serums have high concentrations of active ingredients. Use a serum that is appropriate for your skin type after toning and cleansing.

4. Get enough sleep. Sleep deprivation can result in puffiness, dark circles, and dull skin. For your skin to heal and regenerate, aim for 7-8 hours of sleep each night.

To maintain healthy, radiant skin, it is crucial to establish a daily skincare routine that includes cleansing, toning, and moisturizing. You can keep your skin looking and feeling its best by selecting the best skincare products for your skin type and incorporating extra practices like wearing sunscreen, exfoliating, using serums, and getting enough sleep.

Specific Skin Issues and Their Causes

- Acne
- Rosacea
- Eczema
- Psoriasis
- Aging skin

While using the right skincare products can help maintain healthy, radiant skin, many people have particular skin problems that call for specialized care. In this chapter, we'll talk about a few typical skin problems, their causes, and remedies.

Acne

People of all ages are susceptible to this common skin condition. Acne, blackheads, and whiteheads are the results of the hair follicles becoming clogged with oil and dead skin cells. Acne can be influenced by hormonal changes, stress, diet, and specific medications. Keeping the skin clean and avoiding picking or squeezing pimples are crucial for managing acne. Salicylic acid and benzoyl peroxide-based over-the-counter acne medications can also be beneficial.

Rosacea

Rosacea is a chronic skin ailment that results in facial bumps, flushing, and redness. It is more prevalent in people with fair skin and can be brought on by alcohol, spicy foods, stress, and sun exposure. Avoiding triggers and using gentle skincare products designed for sensitive skin are essential for managing rosacea. In more severe situations, prescription drugs like oral antibiotics or topical creams may also be required.

Eczema

Eczema is a skin condition that causes dry, irritated skin that itches and swells. Allergens, irritants, stress, and temperature changes can all cause it. Regular skin moisturizing is crucial for managing eczema, as is avoiding triggers. In more severe circumstances, prescription drugs like topical steroids or immunomodulators might also be required.

Psoriasis

A chronic skin condition that results in thick, scaly skin patches. Stress, infections, and specific medications can all serve as triggers for it, which is brought on by an overactive immune system. It's crucial to keep the skin moisturized and stay away from triggers in order to manage psoriasis. In more severe circumstances, prescription drugs like systemic or topical steroids might also be required.

Aging skin

As we get older, our skin changes, losing elasticity, producing less collagen, and becoming drier. Wrinkles, fine lines, and age spots may result from these modifications. Protecting the skin from sun damage, moisturizing frequently, and using anti-aging skincare products with ingredients like retinol, vitamin C, and peptides are all crucial for managing aging skin.

In conclusion, there are numerous treatments available to manage specific skin issues, even though they can be difficult to deal with. You can enhance the look and health of your skin by comprehending the underlying causes of each problem and using specific skincare products and treatments.

Treatment Options

- Over-the-counter skincare products
- Prescription medications and treatments
- Natural remedies

We covered some typical skin conditions and their causes in Chapter 3. We will examine the various management strategies for these skin problems in this chapter.

Over-the-counter skincare products

over-the-counter skincare products are widely available and can be used to treat a variety of skin conditions, including acne, dry skin, and aging skin. Active ingredients in these products may include salicylic acid, benzoyl peroxide, retinol, and hyaluronic acid. It's crucial to select skincare products that are right for your skin type and to carefully adhere to the directions.

Prescription drugs and treatments

In some circumstances, it may be necessary to treat skin problems with pre-scription drugs or treatments. Anti-inflammatory drugs may be prescribed for eczema or psoriasis, for instance, or prescription-strength retinoids may be prescribed for severe acne. For some skin conditions, additional therapies like chemical peels, microdermabrasion, and laser therapy may also be advised.

Natural treatments

Many people prefer to treat their skin problems with natural treatments. For instance, aloe vera gel can be used to soothe dry skin, tea tree oil can be used to treat acne, and oatmeal baths can be used to relieve eczema. Natural remedies can be helpful, but it's important to keep in mind that not all of them are safe, effective, or won't irritate your skin.

In conclusion, there are a variety of treatments available to address particular skin problems. Skin problems can be effectively treated with over-the-counter skincare products, prescription drugs and treatments, and home remedies. To get the best results, it's crucial to pick the best course of action for your particular skin problem and to carefully adhere to the directions.

Healthy Eating for Healthy Skin

- Foods that promote healthy skin
- The importance of hydration
- The link between diet and skin issues

Regarding your skin, the adage "you are what you eat" is accurate. Your diet is incredibly important for maintaining beautiful, healthy skin. We will examine the connection between diet and skin health in this chapter and learn about the foods that support healthy skin.

Foods that support healthy skin

Some foods are a good source of vitamins, minerals, and antioxidants that support healthy skin. By including these foods in your diet, you can give your skin the vital nutrients it needs from the inside out. Here are a few instances:

- **Vegetables and fruits:** The vitamins and antioxidants found in berries, citrus fruits, leafy greens, and colorful vegetables help to prevent oxidative stress and encourage the production of collagen.

- **Omega-3 fatty acids:** Rich in omega-3 fatty acids are fatty fish like salmon, mackerel, and sardines as well as chia seeds, flaxseeds, and walnuts.

These fatty acids support skin elasticity maintenance and inflammation reduction.

- **Healthy fats:** Nuts, avocados, and olive oil all contain healthy fats that help to keep the skin moisturized and supple.

Foods high in water content like watermelon, cucumbers, and celery can help hydrate you and promote supple, healthy skin.

The significance of hydration

For healthy skin, hydration is crucial. Maintaining the skin's moisture balance, eliminating toxins, and promoting a radiant complexion are all made easier by drinking enough water. Consuming hydrating foods like watermelon and cucumbers can boost general hydration levels in addition to drinking water.

The connection between diet and skin problems: 3. Skin problems can result from poor dietary habits. For instance:

- **Sugar and refined carbohydrates**: Sugar and refined carbohydrate-rich diets can exacerbate inflammation, which can result in skin conditions like acne and early aging.

- **Dairy products:** Consuming dairy products can cause some people to develop skin conditions like acne. Making informed dietary decisions can be aided by being aware of how your body reacts to dairy.

- **Prepared meals**: Trans fats, additives, and preservative-rich foods can worsen skin conditions by causing more inflammation in the body.

You can enhance the general health and appearance of your skin by consciously choosing to include skin-friendly foods in your diet and minimizing the consumption of foods that may cause skin problems.

In conclusion, eating well is very important for maintaining healthy skin. The nutrients needed to maintain healthy skin can be obtained by eating a balanced diet that is high in fruits, vegetables, omega-3 fatty acids, and healthy fats. Healthy skin can also be attained by drinking plenty of water, avoiding processed foods, and other substances that might irritate the skin. Keep in mind that internal skin nourishment is just as important as external skincare techniques.

Other Factors That Affect Your Skin

- Sun exposure and protection
- Smoking and its effects on skin
- Stress and its impact on skin health

Diet and other lifestyle choices are not the only things that have a big impact on your skin's health and appearance. Three significant factors will be covered in this chapter: stress, smoking, and sun exposure and protection.

Sun exposure and protection

One of the main factors contributing to skin damage and early aging is excessive exposure to the sun's damaging ultraviolet (UV) rays. Long-term sun exposure raises the risk of skin cancer and can cause sunburn, wrinkles, age spots, and even sunburn. Follow these recommendations to protect your skin from the sun:

- **Use sun protection:** Apply liberal amounts of a broad-spectrum sunscreen with a sun protection factor (SPF) of at least 30 to all exposed skin.

- **Seek cover:** Spend as little time as possible in the sun, especially between 10 a.m. and 4 p.m. when the sun's rays are at their strongest.

- **Dress in a protective manner:** To further protect your skin, dress in long sleeved shirts, pants, and wide-brimmed hats.

- **Put on sunglasses Put on UVA and UVB-blocking sunglasses to safeguard your eyes and the sensitive skin around them.**

Smoking's effects on skin

Smoking is bad for your general health, which includes the condition of your skin. Because blood vessels are constricted by the chemicals in cigarette smoke, less blood reaches the skin, depriving it of vital nutrients and oxygen. This may result in a number of skin conditions, such as:

-**Smoking can speed up the aging process by causing fine lines, wrinkles, and dull skin.**

- **Skin discoloration:** Smoking can cause an uneven skin tone and a yellowish complexion.

-**Smoking makes it harder for the skin to heal wounds and bounce back from procedures or injuries.**

- **Increased risk of developing certain types of skin cancer:** Smoking is associated with an increased risk of developing these cancers.

Giving up smoking can have a significant positive impact on your overall health as well as the condition of your skin.

Stress and its effects on skin health

Prolonged stress can cause skin problems and aggravate pre-existing ones. Your body releases cortisol and other stress hormones when you are under stress, which can increase oil production and cause acne breakouts. Stress can also interfere with the skin's normal barrier function, increasing sensitivity and irritability. To control stress and keep skin healthy:

   - **Engage in stress-relieving exercises**: To reduce stress, practice techniques like yoga, deep breathing exercises, meditation, or routine exercise.

   - **Get adequate rest:** Aim for restful sleep because it encourages skin renewal and repair.

   - **Make self-care a priority. Schedule time for enjoyable activities, quality time with loved ones, and pastimes that allow you to unwind.**

Finally, factors like stress, smoking, and sun exposure can have a big impact on the condition and appearance of your skin. You can help to maintain healthier, more youthful skin by using stress-reduction techniques, avoiding smoking, and applying sun protection. Remember that both internal and external factors must be taken into account when caring for your skin.

Skin Care for Different Stages of Life

- Skincare for babies and children
- Skincare for teenagers
- Skincare for pregnant women
- Skincare for menopausal women

Our skin changes in different ways as we go through different stages of life and needs particular care. The topic of skincare considerations for infants, children, teenagers, pregnant women, and menopausal women will be the main focus of this chapter.

Skin care for infants and kids

- **Gentle cleansing:** To properly clean a baby or child's delicate skin, use gentle, fragrance-free cleansers.

- **Moisturization:** To keep their skin hydrated and protected, use a mild, hypoallergenic moisturizer.

- **Sun protection**: Cover their skin with broad-spectrum sunscreen with a high SPF and wear protective clothing, hats, and sunglasses to protect it from the sun's harmful UV rays.

- **Diaper care:** Use diaper creams or ointments to protect and soothe the skin and change diapers frequently to prevent diaper rash.

Teenage skin care

Encourage teenagers to establish a regular cleansing schedule to get rid of extra oil, dirt, and impurities that can exacerbate acne. Use non-comedogenic, gentle cleansers.

- **Acne treatment:** If acne is a problem, you should think about using over-the-counter acne medications with ingredients like salicylic acid or benzoyl peroxide. To avoid scarring, exhort them to refrain from picking or squeezing pimples.

- **Sun protection:** Emphasize the value of sun protection to teenagers and encourage the use of sunscreen to fend off sun damage.

- **Balanced diet:** To support general skin health, encourage a healthy diet rich in fruits, vegetables, and whole grains.

Pregnant women's skincare

- **Gentle skincare products:** To reduce skin sensitivity during pregnancy, choose gentle, fragrance-free skincare products.

- **Stretch mark avoidance:** Apply oils or moisturizers frequently to body parts that are vulnerable to stretch marks, such as the hips, breasts, and abdomen.

- **Sun protection:** Use sunscreen designed for sensitive skin and wear protective clothing to shield the skin from UV rays.

- **Consultation with a medical professional:** Prior to beginning any new skincare regimen or treatment while pregnant, always seek medical advice.

Menopausal women's skin care

- **Hydration:** Give hydrating skincare products and moisturizers top priority because hormonal changes during menopause can result in drier skin.
  - **Sun protection:** Continue to use sunscreen and seek out shade to protect your skin from UV rays.
  - **Anti-aging skincare:** To address issues like wrinkles and loss of elasticity, think about incorporating anti-aging products with components like retinol, peptides, and antioxidants.
  - **Consultation with a dermatologist:** If you notice significant changes in your skin, make an appointment to see a dermatologist for individualized advice and possible treatments.

Finally, different life stages have different skincare requirements. Maintaining healthy and youthful skin can be achieved by adapting skincare routines to each stage, such as using gentle products on infants and young children, addressing teenage acne issues, adjusting for pregnancy, and addressing the effects of menopause. It's critical to comprehend the particular requirements of each stage and, when necessary, to seek professional advice.

Conclusion

This book has covered a variety of skin care topics, from understanding different skin types to treating specific skin problems, forming healthy eating habits, and taking environmental factors that affect skin health into account. Let's review some key ideas as we come to a close to this journey and emphasize the significance of giving skin health top priority.

1. Recognizing your skin type: We talked about the five basic skin types, including normal, oily, dry, combination, and sensitive. We also looked at how to identify your skin type. Knowing your skin type is essential because it helps you select the right skincare products and treatments.

2. The fundamental steps of a daily skincare routine were covered, with a focus on cleansing, moisturizing, and sun protection. You can keep your skin looking healthy and radiant by sticking to a routine and using products that are right for your skin type.

3. Specific skin conditions: We looked at conditions like rosacea, eczema, psoriasis, acne, and aging skin. You can effectively manage these problems and get professional assistance when you need to by being aware of their causes and available treatments.

4. Treatment options: We talked about the various treatment options, such as over-the-counter skincare items, prescribed drugs and treatments, and home remedies. Your skin's health and appearance can change significantly

depending on which treatment option you select for your particular skin problem.

5. A balanced diet full of fruits, vegetables, omega-3 fatty acids, and healthy fats is important for maintaining healthy skin. Skin-friendly diets help to maintain the health and radiance of your skin.

6. External factors: We looked into how stress, smoking, and sun exposure affected skin health. Smoking abstinence, stress management, and sun protection all contribute to healthy skin in general.

Finally, it is critical to give skin health top priority because it not only affects appearance but also reflects general wellbeing. You can achieve and maintain healthy, radiant skin by adhering to the guidelines and suggestions provided in this book. Keep in mind to consistently follow a skincare regimen, pick suitable products, and get expert advice when required.

Encouragement to prioritize skin health

The remarkable organ that is your skin deserves your care and consideration. Making skin health a priority is an investment in your general wellbeing and self-confidence. In addition to being attractive, healthy skin acts as a barrier to protect your body and preserve its health and vitality.

Keep in mind that over time, every action you take to take care of your skin makes a difference. In order to achieve and maintain healthy skin, consistency and patience are essential. Accept the journey, pay attention to your skin's particular requirements, and change your routine as needed.

Remember to practice self-care in addition to skincare. Put hydration first, eat a balanced diet, control your stress, and live a healthy lifestyle. Your skin is a reflection of your overall health, and you can benefit from youthful, glowing skin by making thoughtful decisions.

Let the knowledge you gain enable you to make wise decisions about your skin care as you finish this book. Accept the self-care journey, and may your skin glow with vigor and assurance.

About the Author

Emilia Daniels is a writer on several books such as from From Bump to Bundle: A Comprehensive Guide to Pregnancy and Child Care, several books on marriage and inspirational books

www.ingramcontent.com/pod-product-compliance
Lightning Source LLC
Chambersburg PA
CBHW072344270726
48659CB00023B/2373